Sacred Healing:

Unlocking the Power of Gua Sha for Optimal Health and Wellness

Estrella Ortega & Michael DiCicco

Dear Reader,

As the founders of the Sacred Healing Supply Company, we are honored to share our knowledge and passion for natural wellness with you through the pages of this book.

Gua Sha has been used for centuries as a powerful tool for promoting healing and reducing pain, and we are thrilled to see the growing interest in this ancient healing practice. With "Sacred Healing: Unlocking the Power of Gua Sha for Optimal Health and Wellness," we hope to share our extensive experience and expertise with those seeking a safe, effective, and natural way to improve their health and well-being.

What sets "Sacred Healing" apart is its practical, easy-to-follow approach to Gua Sha. We've broken down the techniques and tools of Gua Sha into simple, easy-to-understand steps, making it accessible to anyone, regardless of their level of experience. Our tips and insights are invaluable for both new and experienced practitioners, and our commitment to safety and caution is a testament to our expertise.

This book is not only a comprehensive guide to Gua Sha but also a celebration of the power of natural healing. Our passion for Gua Sha and natural wellness shines through on every page, and our dedication to helping others achieve optimal health and wellness is at the core of everything we do.

We're excited to share our love of Gua Sha and natural wellness with you, and we hope that this book will inspire you to incorporate this powerful healing practice into your daily routine. With "Sacred Healing" as your guide, you too can experience the transformative benefits of Gua Sha and unlock the power of natural healing.

Michael DiCicco and Estrella Ortega
Founders of Sacred Healing Supply Company

Medical Disclaimer:

The information presented in this book is for educational purposes only and is not intended to be a substitute for professional medical advice, diagnosis, or treatment. The authors of this book are not licensed healthcare providers and do not provide medical advice, diagnosis, or treatment.

If you have a medical condition or are taking medication, please consult with your healthcare provider before using Gua Sha or any other natural therapy. Gua Sha is not a substitute for professional medical treatment and should not be used to replace any medications or treatments prescribed by your healthcare provider.

The Sacred Healing Supply Company and the authors of this book are not responsible for any adverse effects or consequences resulting from the use of Gua Sha or any other natural therapy. Always use Gua Sha safely and with caution, and discontinue use if you experience any adverse reactions or discomfort.

The information presented in this book is based on the authors' personal experiences and research, and is not intended to be a comprehensive guide to Gua Sha or natural health and wellness. It is important to do your own research and consult with a qualified healthcare provider before making any changes to your wellness routine.

By using the information presented in this book, you acknowledge and agree that the authors and the Sacred Healing Supply Company are not liable for any direct or indirect consequences of the use of Gua Sha or any other natural therapy.

Chapter List:

CHAPTER I:

Introduction

Definition of Gua Sha and Its History

Gua Sha is an ancient healing practice that has been used for thousands of years in Traditional Chinese Medicine. The term "Gua Sha" means "scraping" in Chinese, and the technique involves using a smooth-edged tool to gently scrape or rub the skin in a specific pattern.

Gua Sha is also known as "coining," "spooning," or "scraping," depending on the type of tool that is used. Traditionally, a smooth-edged coin or spoon was used, but today Gua Sha tools can be made from a variety of materials, including jade, rose quartz, and stainless steel.

The history of Gua Sha can be traced back to ancient China, where it was used as a form of folk medicine to treat a wide range of ailments. The technique was originally used by traditional healers, who would use a smooth-edged tool to scrape the skin over areas of pain or tension. This was believed to help promote the flow of "qi" (pronounced "chee"), which is the life force energy that flows through the body according to Traditional Chinese Medicine.

Over time, Gua Sha became a popular form of therapy in many parts of Asia, and it is still widely used today by practitioners of Traditional Chinese Medicine. In recent years, Gua Sha has gained popularity in the West as a form of alternative medicine and natural beauty therapy.

In the following chapters, we will explore the many benefits of Gua Sha and how it can be used to promote health and wellness in a variety of ways. Whether you are new to Gua Sha or a seasoned practitioner, this book will provide you with a comprehensive guide to understanding and using this ancient healing practice.

Benefits of Gua Sha

Gua Sha is a powerful healing technique that can provide a wide range of benefits for both physical and emotional health. Here are just a few of the many benefits of Gua Sha:

Pain relief: Gua Sha can help to relieve both acute and chronic pain by promoting blood flow to the affected area and releasing tension in the muscles.

Improved circulation: By stimulating blood flow and lymphatic drainage, Gua Sha can help to improve circulation throughout the body, which can promote healing and reduce inflammation.

Relaxation: Gua Sha can be an incredibly relaxing practice that helps to reduce stress and promote a sense of calm.

Detoxification: By promoting lymphatic drainage, Gua Sha can help to remove toxins from the body, which can have a positive impact on overall health.

Anti-aging: Gua Sha is also becoming increasingly popular as a natural beauty therapy, as it can help to reduce the appearance of wrinkles and promote a more youthful complexion.

These are just a few of the many benefits of Gua Sha. In the following chapters, we will explore these benefits in more detail and provide you with the knowledge and tools you need to start using Gua Sha for yourself.

Different Types of Gua Sha Tools

Gua Sha tools come in a variety of shapes and sizes, each with their own unique benefits and uses. Here are some of the most common types of Gua Sha tools:

Traditional Gua Sha board: This is the most common type of Gua Sha tool and is typically made of jade, rose quartz, or other natural materials. It has a smooth, flat surface and is used to scrape the skin in long strokes to promote circulation and release tension.

Guasha comb: This type of tool has a serrated edge and is used to gently scrape the skin in a comb-like motion. It is particularly effective for treating areas with thicker muscle layers, such as the back and thighs.

Guasha roller: This tool has a rolling head with ridges or bumps that are designed to stimulate the skin and promote blood flow. It is often used on the face to reduce puffiness and promote a more youthful appearance.

Gua Sha spoon: This type of tool has a concave shape and is used to gently press and scrape the skin in specific areas to release tension and promote healing. It is particularly effective for treating acupressure points and meridians.

Metal Gua Sha: This type of tool, like the Sacred Healing Supply Company Gua Sha, is made of metal and has a smooth, flat surface. It is a popular choice for those who prefer a firmer pressure and is often used to treat larger areas of the body, such as the back or legs.

There are many other types of Gua Sha tools available, each with their own unique benefits and uses. In the following chapters, we will explore these tools in more detail and provide you with the knowledge and tools you need to start using Gua Sha for yourself.

CHAPTER II:

Understanding Gua Sha: The Science Behind the Practice

As with any ancient healing practice, Gua Sha is steeped in tradition and folklore. However, as modern science advances, we are discovering more and more about the actual mechanisms behind this powerful technique. At its core, Gua Sha is rooted in the principles of Traditional Chinese Medicine (TCM), a holistic healing system that dates back over 2,000 years.

TCM is based on the belief that the body is a complex network of interconnected systems, and that imbalances or blockages in one area can have far-reaching effects on overall health and wellbeing. Gua Sha is just one of many TCM techniques that are designed to help restore balance and promote healing.

According to TCM principles, the body has a system of channels or pathways known as meridians, which flow through the body and carry energy, or Qi. When the Qi in these meridians becomes blocked or stagnant, it can lead to pain, inflammation, and other health problems.

Gua Sha is thought to work by stimulating the flow of Qi and promoting the movement of stagnant energy. When the skin is scraped with a Gua Sha tool, it creates small, controlled injuries that trigger a healing response in the body. This response includes the release of anti-inflammatory and immune-boosting substances, as well as an increase in circulation and blood flow to the affected area.

In the following chapters, we will dive deeper into the science behind Gua Sha and explore how it can be used to address a wide range of health concerns, from chronic pain to digestive issues and beyond. By understanding the underlying principles of this powerful technique, you can unlock its full potential and tap into the healing power of Traditional Chinese Medicine.

Anatomy and Physiology: The Physical Mechanisms Behind Gua Sha

While the principles of Traditional Chinese Medicine provide a broad framework for understanding Gua Sha, the physical mechanisms behind this technique are equally important to consider. To truly understand the power of Gua Sha, we must look at the anatomy and physiology of the body, and how this ancient practice can influence these systems.

At its core, Gua Sha works by manipulating the soft tissues of the body, including the skin, fascia, and muscles. By scraping these tissues with a specialized tool, Gua Sha can stimulate a wide range of physiological responses, including:

Increased circulation: When the skin is scraped, it creates microtraumas that trigger a response from the body's circulatory system. Blood vessels in the affected area dilate, allowing more blood and oxygen to flow to the tissues. This increased circulation can help to reduce inflammation, promote healing, and alleviate pain.

Release of tension: Gua Sha can help to release tension and tightness in the muscles and fascia. By applying pressure to these tissues, Gua Sha can help to break up adhesions and improve range of motion.

Activation of the lymphatic system: The lymphatic system plays a crucial role in the body's immune response, and Gua Sha can help to activate this system. By stimulating the lymphatic vessels, Gua Sha can help to remove toxins and waste products from the body, boosting overall health and wellbeing.

Modulation of the nervous system: Gua Sha has been shown to have a calming effect on the nervous system, which can help to reduce stress and anxiety. This effect is likely due to the release of endorphins and other neurotransmitters that occur during and after a Gua Sha treatment.

By understanding the anatomy and physiology behind Gua Sha, we can begin to appreciate just how powerful this technique can be. Whether you're dealing with chronic pain, stress, or a host of other health concerns, Gua Sha offers a safe, natural, and effective way to promote healing and wellbeing.

The Effects of Gua Sha on the Body: How This Technique Can Promote Healing and Wellness

Now that we've explored the anatomy and physiology behind Gua Sha, let's take a closer look at the effects that this technique can have on the body. From reducing pain and inflammation to improving immune function, Gua Sha offers a wide range of benefits for both physical and emotional health.

Here are just a few of the many ways that Gua Sha can impact the body:

Reducing pain and inflammation: Gua Sha has been shown to be an effective treatment for a variety of painful conditions, including back pain, neck pain, and headaches. By increasing circulation and releasing tension in the muscles and fascia, Gua Sha can help to alleviate pain and reduce inflammation.

Boosting immune function: Gua Sha has been found to have immune-boosting effects, helping to promote the body's natural defenses against infection and disease. This may be due in part to the fact that Gua Sha stimulates the lymphatic system, which plays a crucial role in the immune response.

Improving sleep: Gua Sha has a calming effect on the nervous system, which can help to improve sleep quality. By reducing stress and promoting relaxation, Gua Sha can help to support healthy sleep patterns.

Enhancing skin health: Gua Sha can help to improve the appearance and health of the skin, by increasing circulation and promoting lymphatic drainage. This can help to reduce puffiness, minimize fine lines and wrinkles, and promote a healthy glow.

Supporting emotional wellbeing: Gua Sha can have a powerful impact on emotional health, by promoting relaxation and reducing stress. By allowing the body and mind to unwind, Gua Sha can help to promote a sense of calm and wellbeing.

Overall, the effects of Gua Sha on the body are wide-ranging and multifaceted. Whether you're dealing with a specific health concern or simply looking to promote overall wellness, Gua Sha offers a safe and effective way to support your body's natural healing processes.

Preparing for a Gua Sha Session

Before you begin your Gua Sha practice, it's important to properly prepare yourself and your environment to ensure a safe and effective session. In this chapter, we'll cover the steps you should take to prepare for a Gua Sha session, including everything from setting up your space to preparing your body and mind.

Here's an overview of what we'll cover in Chapter III:

1. Setting the Stage: Creating a Peaceful and Relaxing Environment
- How to create a calm and quiet space for your Gua Sha practice
- The role of aromatherapy, music, and other sensory experiences in enhancing your session
- Tips for minimizing distractions and creating a meditative atmosphere

2. Preparing Your Body: Tips and Techniques for Optimizing Your Gua Sha Session
- The role of hydration, diet, and other lifestyle factors in preparing your body for Gua Sha

- How to stretch and warm up your muscles to enhance the effects of Gua Sha
- The importance of proper breathing and relaxation techniques for maximizing the benefits of your session

3. Understanding Your Skin and Sensitivities: How to Avoid Irritation or Injury
- The importance of understanding your skin type and any potential sensitivities or allergies to oils or other lubricants
- How to properly cleanse and prep your skin for Gua Sha
- Tips for avoiding common mistakes that can lead to irritation or injury during your session

4. Choosing the Right Tools: An Overview of Gua Sha Instruments and Accessories
- Overview of different types of Gua Sha tools and how to choose the right one for your needs
- How to properly clean and care for your tools to ensure longevity and optimal performance
- Tips for accessorizing your Gua Sha practice with complementary tools and products, such as jade rollers or gua sha oils

By the end of this chapter, you'll be fully prepared to begin your Gua Sha practice with confidence and ease, knowing that you have taken the necessary steps to create a safe and effective environment for this transformative technique.

Setting the Stage - Creating a Peaceful and Relaxing Environment

Gua Sha is a practice that is all about relaxation and letting go of tension in the body. To fully experience the benefits of this practice, it's important to create a peaceful and relaxing environment that allows you to fully engage with the practice. Here are some tips to help you create the perfect environment for your Gua Sha session:

1. Choose a quiet, calm space: Find a space in your home where you can be undisturbed for the duration of your session. It's important to minimize distractions as much as possible so that you can fully focus on the practice. If you have pets or live with others, let them know ahead of time that you'll be practicing Gua Sha and ask them not to disturb you.

2. Adjust the lighting: The right lighting can make a big difference in creating a peaceful and relaxing environment. You can use soft, warm lighting to create a cozy atmosphere or dim the lights to create a calming ambiance. Avoid bright or harsh lighting, which can be distracting and interfere with relaxation.

3. Use aromatherapy: Essential oils and candles can be a powerful tool in enhancing the sensory experience of your Gua Sha session. Choose scents that promote relaxation, such as lavender or chamomile. You can also experiment with other essential oils that promote relaxation, such as bergamot, clary sage, and ylang-ylang. Aromatherapy can help to soothe the mind and body, and create a sense of calm.

4. Play calming music: Music can be a powerful tool in setting the mood and promoting relaxation. Choose music that is calming and peaceful, and avoid music with distracting or jarring elements. Classical music, nature sounds, or relaxing instrumental music can be good choices. You can also experiment with binaural beats or other types of music that are specifically designed to promote relaxation.

5. Use comfortable pillows and blankets: During your Gua Sha session, you'll be lying down or sitting in a relaxed position for an extended period of time. It's important to be comfortable during this time, so use pillows and blankets to create a cozy and relaxing space. You can also use an eye mask or other props to help you fully relax.

By taking the time to create a peaceful and relaxing environment, you'll be better able to let go of stress, tension, and negative thoughts, allowing you to fully engage with the practice of Gua Sha. The more relaxed and comfortable you are, the more you'll be able to benefit from this powerful practice.

Preparing Your Body: Tips and Techniques for Optimizing Your Gua Sha Session

To get the most out of your Gua Sha session, it's important to prepare your body beforehand. Here are some tips and techniques to help you do that:

1. The role of hydration, diet, and other lifestyle factors: Proper hydration and nutrition are key to supporting

your body's natural healing processes, and can have a big impact on the effectiveness of your Gua Sha session. Before your session, make sure you're drinking enough water to keep your body hydrated and eliminate toxins. Avoid alcohol, caffeine, and heavy meals, which can interfere with the detoxification process and make it harder for your body to process the benefits of Gua Sha. Eating a healthy, balanced meal with plenty of fresh fruits and vegetables can help ensure that your body has the nutrients it needs to support healing and rejuvenation.

2. How to stretch and warm up your muscles: Stretching and warming up your muscles before your Gua Sha session can help enhance its effects. This is especially important if you've been sitting or standing in one position for a long period of time, as it can help loosen up tight muscles and increase circulation. Try doing some gentle stretches or a light workout to get your blood flowing and loosen up your muscles. This can help increase circulation and prepare your body for the Gua Sha session.

3. The importance of proper breathing and relaxation techniques: Gua Sha is a relaxing and therapeutic practice, and it's important to approach it with a calm and focused mindset. Taking a few deep breaths before your session can help quiet your mind and reduce stress, allowing you to fully relax and get the most out of your session. During your Gua Sha session, focus on your breathing and try to let go of any tension or stress in your body. This can help improve the overall effectiveness of your session and enhance your sense of well-being.

4. Other techniques to enhance your Gua Sha session: In addition to the tips above, there are a few other techniques you can use to optimize the effects of your Gua Sha session. For example, you may want to apply a warm compress to the area you'll be working on to help loosen up tight muscles and improve circulation. Massaging the area with a gentle, circular motion can also help increase blood flow and enhance the effects of Gua Sha.

By taking the time to properly prepare your body and mind, you can optimize the effects of your Gua Sha session and experience the full benefits of this ancient healing practice.

Understanding Your Skin and Sensitivities: How to Avoid Irritation or Injury

When it comes to Gua Sha, it's important to take care of your skin to avoid any potential irritation or injury during your session. Understanding your skin type and any potential sensitivities or allergies to oils or other lubricants is crucial. In this section, we'll discuss how to properly cleanse and prep your skin for Gua Sha and provide tips for avoiding common mistakes that can lead to irritation or injury during your session.

1. Understanding Your Skin Type and Sensitivities

The first step in avoiding irritation or injury during your Gua Sha session is understanding your skin type and any potential sensitivities or allergies to oils or other lubricants. If you have sensitive skin, it's important to choose a lubricant that is gentle and non-irritating. For example, you might consider using a fragrance-free oil or a hypoallergenic lotion.

2. How to Properly Cleanse and Prep Your Skin

Properly cleansing and prepping your skin is an important step in preparing for your Gua Sha session. You should start by washing your face with a gentle cleanser to remove any dirt, oil, or makeup. After cleansing, you can apply a toner to help balance your skin's pH levels and prepare it for the Gua Sha session. You can also apply a small amount of lubricant to the area you'll be working on to help the tool glide smoothly over your skin.

3. Tips for Avoiding Common Mistakes

During your Gua Sha session, it's important to be mindful of your movements and avoid common mistakes that can lead to irritation or injury. One common mistake is using too much pressure, which can cause redness, bruising, or even broken capillaries. Another mistake is using the wrong tool or using it improperly, which can cause discomfort or pain. It's important to choose the right tool for your skin type and use it properly by following the instructions or seeking guidance from a professional.

In addition to these tips, it's also important to be mindful of your own body and to listen to any signals it may be sending you. If you experience any discomfort or pain during your Gua Sha session, it's important to stop and assess the situation. You may need to adjust your technique or take a break to allow your skin to recover.

By understanding your skin type, properly cleansing and prepping your skin, and avoiding common mistakes, you can help ensure a safe and effective Gua Sha session.

Choosing the Right Tools: An Overview of Gua Sha Instruments and Accessories

In addition to preparing your body and skin, choosing the right Gua Sha tools and accessories is also an important consideration for a successful Gua Sha session. Here's what you need to know about Gua Sha tools and how to choose the right ones for your needs.

Overview of Different Types of Gua Sha Tools

There are many different types of Gua Sha tools available, ranging from traditional jade and metal scrapers to modern tools made from materials like rose quartz or stainless steel. Some popular types of Gua Sha tools include:

- Traditional jade or horn scrapers: These are the most common and traditional types of Gua Sha tools, made from natural materials and available in a variety of shapes and sizes. Jade is a popular choice due to its cooling properties, while horn scrapers are favored for their durability.
- Metal scrapers: These are typically made from stainless steel and are designed to be used with lubricants like Gua Sha oils to glide smoothly over the skin.

- Rose quartz or other crystal scrapers: These are becoming increasingly popular due to their purported healing and energizing properties, as well as their attractive appearance.
- Electric or battery-powered tools: These are modern versions of traditional Gua Sha tools and use vibration or other technologies to enhance the effects of the massage.

Choosing the Right Gua Sha Tools for Your Needs

When choosing a Gua Sha tool, it's important to consider your personal preferences, as well as the intended use of the tool. Here are some tips to keep in mind:

- Consider the material: Different materials may have different properties or effects on the skin, so it's important to choose one that you feel comfortable with.
- Look for a comfortable grip: Gua Sha tools should be easy to hold and use without slipping, so look for one that feels comfortable in your hand.
- Choose the right size and shape: Depending on the area of the body you are targeting, you may want to choose a tool with a specific shape or size to make it easier to use.
- Consider additional features: Some Gua Sha tools come with additional features, such as rollers or extra attachments, so consider what features you may need or want.

Proper Care and Maintenance of Gua Sha Tools

To ensure the longevity and optimal performance of your Gua Sha tools, it's important to take good care of them. Here are some tips for proper care and maintenance:

- Clean your tools after each use: Use soap and water or a disinfectant to clean your Gua Sha tools after each use, and make sure to dry them thoroughly.
- Store your tools properly: Keep your Gua Sha tools in a clean, dry place, and avoid exposing them to extreme temperatures or moisture.
- Replace your tools as needed: Over time, Gua Sha tools may become worn or damaged, so it's important to replace them as needed to ensure that they continue to work effectively.

Tips for Accessorizing Your Gua Sha Practice

In addition to Gua Sha tools, there are other accessories and products that can enhance your Gua Sha practice. Here are some popular options to consider:

- Gua Sha oils: These lubricants are designed to help the Gua Sha tool glide smoothly over the skin and may also have additional benefits for the skin.
- Jade rollers: These tools are designed to be used in conjunction with Gua Sha and can help to reduce inflammation and puffiness in the skin.

- Facial cups: These small cups are designed to be used on the face and can help to promote circulation and lymphatic drainage.

By choosing the right Gua Sha tools and accessories and taking good care of them, you can maximize the benefits of your Gua Sha practice and enjoy

CHAPTER IV

Performing Gua Sha: Techniques for Different Areas of the Body

Gua Sha is a therapeutic technique that involves using a smooth-edged tool to scrape the skin in order to improve circulation, reduce pain, and promote overall health and well-being. This ancient Chinese healing practice is becoming increasingly popular in Western cultures as more people discover its benefits for the mind, body, and spirit.

In this chapter, we'll explore the techniques for performing Gua Sha on different areas of the body, including the back, neck and shoulders, face, limbs, and abdomen. Each area of the body requires a slightly different technique, and understanding the proper way to perform Gua Sha on each area can help you to maximize its benefits.

Gua Sha for the Back

Gua Sha for the back is an effective way to alleviate pain and tension, as well as improve circulation and promote healing. To perform Gua Sha on the back, it's best to work in sections, starting at the base of the spine and moving upward toward the shoulders. Apply lubricant to the skin, and then use long, firm strokes with your Gua Sha tool, moving in one direction only. Be careful not to apply too much pressure or use a tool that is too sharp, as this can cause bruising or injury.

When performing Gua Sha on the back, it's important to pay attention to the specific areas of tension and focus on those areas in particular. For example, if you have tension in your lower back, you may want to focus on that area first and then work your way up toward the shoulders.

Gua Sha for the Neck and Shoulders

The neck and shoulders are common areas of tension and pain, and Gua Sha can be a great way to relieve these symptoms. To perform Gua Sha on the neck and shoulders, start by applying lubricant to the skin, and then use your Gua Sha tool to make long, sweeping strokes up and down the neck and across the shoulders. Be gentle and avoid applying too much pressure, especially around the delicate areas of the neck.

One effective technique for performing Gua Sha on the neck and shoulders is to use a combination of long, sweeping strokes and smaller, more targeted strokes. This can help to release tension and promote relaxation in the muscles.

Gua Sha for the Face

Gua Sha can also be used on the face to improve circulation, reduce puffiness, and promote a healthy, youthful appearance. To perform Gua Sha on the face, it's best to use a tool with a small, smooth edge, such as a jade roller or a gua sha stone. Apply a small amount of lubricant to the skin, and then use gentle, sweeping strokes to massage the skin. Be careful not to apply too much pressure or use a tool that is too sharp, as this can cause irritation or injury.

When performing Gua Sha on the face, it's important to pay attention to the specific areas of tension and focus on those areas in particular. For example, if you have tension in your jawline, you may want to focus on that area first and then work your way up toward the forehead.

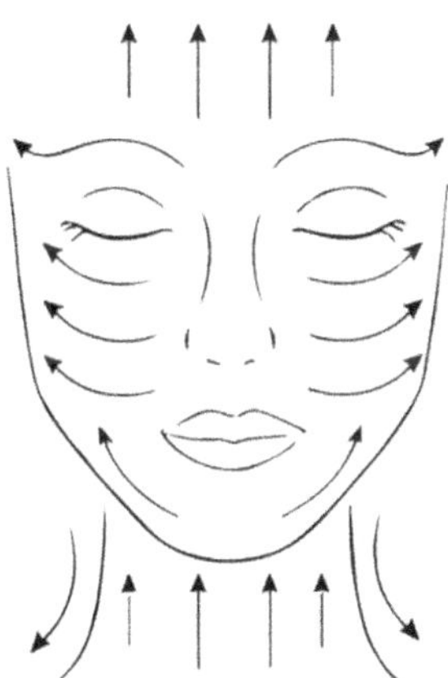

Gua Sha for the Limbs

Gua Sha can be performed on the limbs to improve circulation, reduce pain and tension, and promote healing. To perform Gua Sha on the limbs, it's best to work in sections, starting at the base of the limb and moving upward. Apply lubricant to the skin, and then use long, firm strokes with your Gua Sha tool, moving in one direction only. Be careful not to apply too much pressure or use a tool that is too sharp, as this can cause bruising or injury.

One effective technique for performing Gua Sha on the limbs is to use a combination of long, firm strokes and shorter, more targeted strokes. This can help to release tension and promote relaxation in the muscles.

When performing Gua Sha on the limbs, it's important to pay attention to the specific areas of tension and focus on those areas in particular. For example, if you have tension in your calf muscles, you may want to focus on that area first and then work your way up toward the thigh.

Gua Sha for the Abdomen

Gua Sha for the abdomen can help to improve digestion, reduce bloating and inflammation, and promote overall health and well-being. To perform Gua Sha on the abdomen, start by applying lubricant to the skin, and then use your Gua Sha tool to make gentle, circular motions around the belly button. Be careful not to apply too much pressure, especially around the sensitive organs of the abdomen.

One effective technique for performing Gua Sha on the abdomen is to use a combination of circular motions and targeted strokes in specific areas of tension or pain. This can help to release tension and promote relaxation in the muscles.

When performing Gua Sha on the abdomen, it's important to pay attention to any areas of pain or discomfort, as well as any potential sensitivities or allergies to oils or other lubricants.

By using these techniques for different areas of the body, you can optimize the effects of your Gua Sha practice and promote overall health and well-being. Remember to always use proper technique, be gentle and avoid using too much pressure, and listen to your body to ensure that your Gua Sha practice is safe and effective.

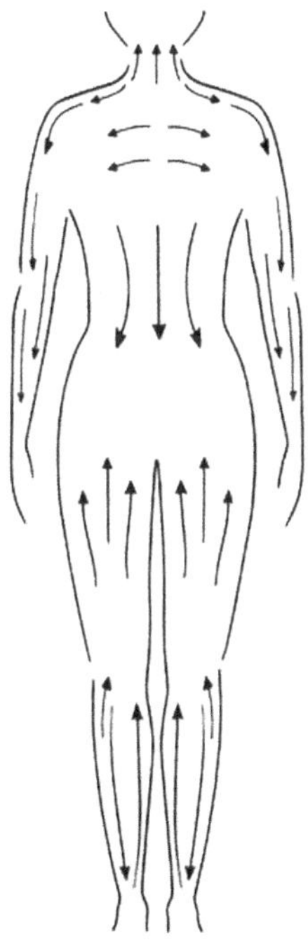

CHAPTER V

Safety and Precautions

Gua Sha is a powerful healing practice that has been used for centuries to promote circulation, reduce pain and inflammation, and promote overall health and well-being. While it is generally considered safe and effective, it's important to take necessary precautions to ensure that your Gua Sha practice is safe, effective, and free from adverse reactions.

In this chapter, we'll explore some of the key safety considerations and best practices for performing Gua Sha, including contraindications, best practices for safety and hygiene, and how to identify and manage adverse reactions.

Contraindications

While Gua Sha is generally safe for most people, there are some contraindications that may make it unsafe or unsuitable for certain individuals. It is important to take these contraindications seriously in order to avoid potential harm or injury. Some of the contraindications include:

- Bleeding disorders or use of blood-thinning medications: If you have a bleeding disorder, such as hemophilia, or are taking blood-thinning medications, you may be at increased risk of bleeding or bruising during a Gua Sha session. If you have any concerns, speak with your healthcare provider before attempting Gua Sha.

- Skin conditions, such as eczema or psoriasis: If you have any skin conditions that cause open sores or lesions, it is best to avoid Gua Sha as it may exacerbate these conditions.

- Open wounds or cuts: If you have any open wounds or cuts, it is best to avoid Gua Sha as it may lead to further injury or infection.

- Varicose veins or broken capillaries: If you have varicose veins or broken capillaries, Gua Sha may cause further damage or injury to these areas.

- Pregnancy: If you are pregnant, it is best to avoid Gua Sha as it may cause contractions or other complications.

- Cancer or other serious illnesses: If you have a serious illness, such as cancer, or are undergoing treatment for a serious illness, it is best to avoid Gua Sha as it may cause further complications or interfere with your treatment.

- Recent surgeries or injuries: If you have had recent surgery or injury, it is best to avoid Gua Sha as it may impede the healing process or cause further injury.

- Fever or acute illness: If you are experiencing a fever or other acute illness, it is best to avoid Gua Sha as it may exacerbate your symptoms.

If you have any of these contraindications, it's important to speak with your healthcare provider before attempting Gua Sha.

Best Practices for Safety and Hygiene

To ensure a safe and hygienic Gua Sha experience, it's important to follow these best practices:

- Use a clean, sterile Gua Sha tool or one that has been properly sanitized before use: It is important to use a clean, sanitized tool to avoid the spread of germs or bacteria.
- Use lubricant or oil to prevent irritation or injury to the skin: Lubricant or oil can help to prevent irritation or injury to the skin during a Gua Sha session.
- Be gentle and avoid using too much pressure, especially on sensitive areas of the body: It is important to be gentle during a Gua Sha session to avoid injury or pain.
- Use proper technique and avoid using a tool that is too sharp or rough: Proper technique is important to ensure a safe and effective Gua Sha session.
- Avoid performing Gua Sha on areas of the body that are swollen, inflamed, or painful: It is best to avoid areas of the body that are swollen, inflamed, or painful to avoid further injury or discomfort.

- Always clean and sanitize your Gua Sha tool after use to prevent the spread of germs or bacteria: Cleaning and sanitizing your Gua Sha tool after each use is important to avoid the spread of germs or bacteria.

Adverse Reactions and How to Manage Them

In rare cases, Gua Sha can cause adverse reactions, such as bruising, skin irritation, or pain. If you experience any adverse reactions during or after a Gua Sha session, it's important to take the following steps:

- Stop the Gua Sha session immediately: If you experience any adverse reactions during a Gua Sha session, stop the session immediately to avoid further injury or discomfort.
- Apply ice to the affected area to reduce swelling and pain: Applying ice to the affected area can help to reduce swelling and pain.
- If the bruising or pain persists, speak with your healthcare provider: If the bruising or pain persists for more than a few days, it's important to speak with your healthcare provider to ensure that there are no underlying health issues or concerns.

It's also important to listen to your body during a Gua Sha session and to communicate with your Gua Sha practitioner if you experience any discomfort or pain. A skilled practitioner will be able to adjust the pressure and technique to ensure a safe and effective Gua Sha experience.

Conclusion

By following these safety considerations and best practices for hygiene and technique, you can ensure a safe and positive Gua Sha experience and reap the many benefits of this ancient healing practice. Remember to always listen to your body, be gentle and avoid using too much pressure, and communicate with your healthcare provider if you have any concerns or questions about the safety of Gua Sha. With proper care and attention, Gua Sha can be a safe and effective way to promote circulation, reduce pain and inflammation, and promote overall health and well-being.

CHAPTER VI

Gua Sha for Pain Relief

Gua Sha is a powerful therapeutic technique that has been used for centuries to relieve pain and promote healing in the body. In this chapter, we'll explore the ways in which Gua Sha can be used for pain relief in greater detail, including how it works, case studies and testimonials, and techniques for common types of pain.

How Gua Sha Helps with Pain

Gua Sha works by stimulating circulation and promoting the flow of Qi, or vital energy, throughout the body. When performed correctly, Gua Sha can help to release tension and blockages in the muscles and connective tissues, reducing pain and promoting healing.

Research has shown that Gua Sha is effective at reducing pain in a variety of conditions, including:

- Neck pain
- Low back pain

- Plantar fasciitis
- Carpal tunnel syndrome
- Fibromyalgia
- Headaches
- Arthritis

In addition to its effects on circulation and Qi flow, Gua Sha has been shown to have a number of other therapeutic benefits, including:

- Reducing inflammation: Gua Sha can help to reduce inflammation in the body, which can be a major contributor to pain and discomfort. Inflammation can occur in response to injury or overuse of a particular area of the body and can be particularly problematic in chronic conditions such as arthritis.
- Promoting relaxation: Gua Sha can help to promote relaxation and reduce stress, which can also contribute to pain relief. Stress can cause tension and tightness in the muscles, which can exacerbate pain and discomfort.
- Stimulating the immune system: Gua Sha has been shown to stimulate the immune system, which can help to promote healing and reduce pain. When the immune system is functioning properly, it can help to reduce inflammation and prevent the development of chronic conditions.

Case Studies and Testimonials

Numerous case studies and testimonials have demonstrated the effectiveness of Gua Sha for pain relief. For example, a study (1) of 40 patients with chronic low back pain found that those who received Gua Sha treatments experienced significant reductions in pain and improved mobility, compared to those who received conventional physical therapy. The study concluded that Gua Sha is a safe and effective treatment option for chronic low back pain.

Another study (2) of 20 patients with neck pain found that Gua Sha was effective at reducing pain and improving range of motion, with results lasting for up to three months after treatment. The study also found that Gua Sha was well-tolerated by patients and did not cause any adverse reactions.

Techniques for Common Types of Pain

Gua Sha can be used to relieve pain in a variety of areas of the body, including the back, neck, shoulders, limbs, and abdomen. Here are some techniques for common types of pain:

- Back pain: Gua Sha can be used to relieve back pain by focusing on the muscles and connective tissues around the spine. A skilled practitioner may use a combination of long, sweeping strokes and targeted strokes to release tension and promote healing in the affected area.

- Neck and shoulder pain: Gua Sha can be used to relieve tension and pain in the neck and shoulder area by focusing on the muscles around the base of the skull and the tops of the shoulders. A practitioner may use a combination of short, targeted strokes and circular motions to release tension and promote relaxation in these areas.

- Limb pain: Gua Sha can be used to relieve pain in the arms and legs by focusing on the muscles and connective tissues in the affected area. A practitioner may use a combination of long, sweeping strokes and targeted strokes to release tension and promote healing.

- Abdominal pain: Gua Sha can be used to relieve abdominal pain by focusing on the muscles and connective tissues around the belly button. A practitioner may use gentle, circular motions to promote circulation and reduce inflammation in the area.

- In addition to these techniques, a skilled Gua Sha practitioner will be able to tailor the treatment to your individual needs and conditions. They may also recommend other complementary therapies, such as acupuncture, massage, or herbal remedies, to further enhance the effects of Gua Sha.

- Safety and Precautions

- While Gua Sha is generally considered safe and well-tolerated, there are some precautions that should be taken to ensure a safe and effective treatment. For example, it's important to avoid areas of the body where there is thin skin or where bones are close to the surface, such as the spine or the shins. It's also important to use a light touch and to avoid applying too much pressure, as this can lead to bruising or other adverse reactions.

- If you have any underlying health conditions or concerns, it's important to speak with your healthcare provider before beginning a Gua Sha treatment. They can help you determine whether Gua Sha is a safe and appropriate treatment option for your individual needs.

- Conclusion
- Gua Sha is a safe, effective, and non-invasive way to relieve pain and promote healing in the body. By working with a skilled practitioner and following proper technique and safety considerations, you can experience the many benefits of this ancient healing practice and improve your quality of life. Whether you are suffering from chronic pain or acute discomfort, Gua Sha can be an excellent way to alleviate symptoms and promote overall health and well-being. With proper care and attention, Gua Sha can help you live a happier, healthier life.

Sacred Healing Supply Company's Gua Sha tool is also an excellent choice for pain relief. Its smooth, curved edges make it easy to use on the skin without causing discomfort, and the high-quality stainless steel construction ensures durability and long-lasting use. The tool can be used to gently scrape and massage the skin, promoting blood flow and lymphatic drainage to reduce inflammation and alleviate pain in the affected area. Whether you're dealing with chronic pain or acute discomfort from an injury, the Sacred Healing Supply Company Gua Sha tool can help to alleviate your symptoms and promote healing in the body.

1- Lauche, R., Materdey, S., Cramer, H., Haller, H., Stange, R., & Dobos, G. (2017). Effectiveness of home-based cupping massage compared to progressive muscle relaxation in patients with chronic neck pain-A randomized controlled trial. PloS one, 12(2), e0171721.

2- Braun, M., Schwickert, M., Nielsen, A., Brunnhuber, S., & Dobos, G. (2011). Effectiveness of traditional Chinese "gua sha" therapy in patients with chronic neck pain: a randomized controlled trial. Pain Medicine, 12(3), 362-369.

CHAPTER VII:

Gua Sha for Skin Health

Gua Sha is an effective therapy not just for pain relief, but also for improving the health and appearance of the skin. In this chapter, we'll explore the benefits of Gua Sha for the skin, as well as techniques for facial rejuvenation and improving skin health on other parts of the body.

Benefits for the Skin

Gua Sha can help to improve the health and appearance of the skin in several ways. Some of the benefits of Gua Sha for the skin include:

- Improving circulation: Gua Sha promotes blood flow and lymphatic drainage, which can help to bring vital nutrients and oxygen to the skin cells. Improved circulation can also help to reduce inflammation and puffiness in the skin.

- Increasing collagen production: Gua Sha can stimulate the production of collagen, which is a key component of healthy, youthful-looking skin. Collagen helps to support the structure of the skin and keep it firm and supple.

- Reducing wrinkles and fine lines: By stimulating circulation and increasing collagen production, Gua Sha can help to reduce the appearance of wrinkles and fine lines in the skin.

- Improving skin tone and texture: Gua Sha can help to improve the tone and texture of the skin by promoting cell regeneration and reducing inflammation. The result is smoother, brighter, and more even-looking skin.

Techniques for Facial Rejuvenation

Gua Sha can be used to promote facial rejuvenation and improve the overall health and appearance of the skin on the face. Here are some techniques for using Gua Sha on the face:

- Start with a clean, dry face: Before beginning a Gua Sha treatment on the face, it's important to start with a clean, dry surface. You can use a gentle cleanser and toner to remove any dirt, oil, or makeup.

- Apply a facial oil or serum: To help the Gua Sha tool glide smoothly over the skin, it's important to use a facial oil or serum. You can use a product specifically designed for Gua Sha, or choose a high-quality, natural oil like jojoba or argan oil.

- Use gentle, upward strokes: When using Gua Sha on the face, it's important to use gentle, upward strokes to promote circulation and lymphatic drainage. Start at the center of the face and work your way outward, using light pressure and a slow, deliberate motion.

- Focus on problem areas: If you have specific areas of concern on your face, such as wrinkles or dark circles, you can spend extra time using Gua Sha in those areas. Use a more targeted approach, using smaller, circular motions to promote circulation and increase collagen production.

- Finish with a cooling tool: After using Gua Sha on the face, you can finish with a cooling tool like a jade roller or a chilled facial stone. This can help to reduce inflammation and puffiness, leaving your skin feeling refreshed and revitalized.

Techniques for Improving Skin Health on Other Parts of the Body

Gua Sha can also be used to improve the health and appearance of the skin on other parts of the body. Here are some techniques for using Gua Sha on other parts of the body:

- Start with a lubricant: Before using Gua Sha on other parts of the body, it's important to apply a lubricant like oil or lotion. This will help the Gua Sha tool glide smoothly over the skin, reducing the risk of irritation or injury.

- Use gentle, sweeping strokes: When using Gua Sha on other parts of the body, use gentle, sweeping strokes to promote circulation and reduce tension in the muscles and connective tissues. Focus on problem areas or areas of tension, using more targeted strokes as needed.

- Experiment with different tools: Gua Sha can be performed using a variety of tools, including jade, rose quartz, and metal. Each type of tool offers its own unique benefits and can be used to target different areas of the body. The Sacred Healing Supply Company Gua Sha tool, for example, is made from high-quality stainless steel and is designed to provide gentle yet effective pressure on the skin. Its ergonomic shape and smooth edges make it easy to use and comfortable to hold, even during longer sessions.

Overall, Gua Sha is an effective and non-invasive way to promote skin health and rejuvenation. By using the right techniques and tools, you can improve circulation, boost collagen production, and reduce inflammation and puffiness in the skin. Whether you are focusing on the face or other parts of the body, Gua Sha can be a powerful tool for achieving healthier, more radiant skin.

CHAPTER VIII:

Gua Sha for Detoxification

Gua Sha is a powerful therapy for promoting detoxification in the body. In this chapter, we'll explore how Gua Sha helps with detoxification, as well as techniques for promoting lymphatic drainage and circulation. We'll also discuss why the Sacred Healing Supply Company's Gua Sha tool is the perfect choice for detoxification and promoting optimal health.

How Gua Sha Helps with Detoxification

Gua Sha helps with detoxification in several ways. First, it promotes lymphatic drainage, which helps to remove toxins and waste products from the body. Lymphatic drainage is an important process that allows the body to eliminate waste and maintain optimal health. By promoting lymphatic drainage, Gua Sha helps to improve the function of the lymphatic system and remove waste products that can build up in the body.

Gua Sha also helps with detoxification by promoting circulation. When the blood and lymphatic systems are working properly, they can effectively remove toxins and waste products from the body.

Gua Sha promotes circulation by increasing blood flow to the affected area, which can help to remove toxins and promote healing.

Techniques for Promoting Lymphatic Drainage

To promote lymphatic drainage with Gua Sha, it's important to use the right techniques. Here are some tips for promoting lymphatic drainage with Gua Sha:

- Start with a lubricant: Before using Gua Sha, it's important to apply a lubricant like oil or lotion to the skin. This will help the Gua Sha tool glide smoothly over the skin and reduce the risk of irritation or injury.
- Use light, sweeping strokes: When using Gua Sha for lymphatic drainage, it's important to use light, sweeping strokes that follow the natural direction of lymphatic flow. This will help to move lymphatic fluid out of the affected area and promote drainage.
- Focus on problem areas: If you have specific areas of concern, such as swollen lymph nodes or areas of inflammation, you can focus your Gua Sha treatment on those areas to promote lymphatic drainage.

Techniques for Promoting Circulation

To promote circulation with Gua Sha, it's important to use the right techniques. Here are some tips for promoting circulation with Gua Sha:

- Start with a lubricant: As with lymphatic drainage, it's important to apply a lubricant like oil or lotion to the skin before using Gua Sha for circulation. This will help the tool glide smoothly over the skin and reduce the risk of irritation or injury.

- Use gentle, sweeping strokes: When using Gua Sha for circulation, use gentle, sweeping strokes to promote blood flow to the affected area. The goal is to promote circulation without causing discomfort or irritation.

- Focus on problem areas: If you have specific areas of concern, such as areas of inflammation or poor circulation, you can focus your Gua Sha treatment on those areas to promote circulation.

Why the Sacred Healing Supply Company's Gua Sha Tool is Perfect

The Sacred Healing Supply Company's Gua Sha tool is the perfect choice for promoting detoxification and optimal health. Its smooth, curved edges make it easy to use on the skin without causing discomfort, and the high-quality stainless steel construction ensures durability and long-lasting use. The tool can be used to gently scrape and massage the skin, promoting lymphatic drainage and circulation to reduce inflammation and promote detoxification. Its ergonomic shape and smooth edges make it easy to use and comfortable to hold, even during longer sessions. Whether you're looking to promote lymphatic drainage, circulation, or detoxification, the Sacred Healing Supply Company's Gua Sha tool is a reliable and effective choice for improving your health and well-being.

CHAPTER IX

Gua Sha for Respiratory Health

Gua Sha is a natural and non-invasive therapy that can help improve respiratory health and alleviate respiratory symptoms. This chapter will delve into the many benefits of Gua Sha for the respiratory system, the techniques used to promote respiratory health with Gua Sha, and how the Sacred Healing Supply Company's Gua Sha tool can be used to improve respiratory health.

Benefits for the Respiratory System

Gua Sha can provide a range of benefits for the respiratory system, which include reducing inflammation, promoting lymphatic drainage, and relieving tension. Reducing inflammation in the respiratory system can result in improved breathing and a decrease in respiratory symptoms such as wheezing or coughing. Lymphatic drainage can remove excess fluid and waste from the lungs and airways, which promotes better respiratory function. By using Gua Sha to relieve tension in the muscles and connective tissues around the respiratory system, it can improve breathing and reduce discomfort.

Techniques for Promoting Respiratory Health

Gua Sha can be used to promote respiratory health by using specific techniques. To promote respiratory health with Gua Sha, follow these tips:

- Start with a lubricant: Using a lubricant such as oil or lotion is essential before using Gua Sha. This will help the tool glide smoothly over the skin and reduce the risk of skin irritation or injury.
- Use gentle, sweeping strokes: Using gentle, sweeping strokes promotes lymphatic drainage and reduces tension in the muscles and connective tissues surrounding the respiratory system.
- Focus on specific areas: For people with congestion in the chest or discomfort in the throat, focusing on these areas will provide greater benefits to the respiratory system.

Using the Sacred Healing Supply Company's Gua Sha Tool to Improve Respiratory Health

The Sacred Healing Supply Company's Gua Sha tool is a great choice to improve respiratory health. The tool's smooth, curved edges allow for easy use without causing discomfort or irritation, and its high-quality stainless steel construction ensures longevity and optimal performance. By using the tool to gently scrape and massage the skin, it promotes lymphatic drainage and reduces tension in the muscles and connective tissues around the respiratory system, improving breathing and reducing discomfort. The ergonomic shape and smooth edges make it comfortable to hold during longer sessions. By incorporating the Sacred Healing Supply Company's Gua Sha tool into your daily self-care routine, you can improve your respiratory health and enjoy better breathing.

If you suffer from respiratory issues, the Sacred Healing Supply Company's Gua Sha tool can be a natural and effective way to alleviate respiratory symptoms, promote respiratory health, and improve breathing. By using the right techniques and incorporating Gua Sha into your daily routine, you can enjoy better respiratory health and improve your overall well-being.

CHAPTER X

Gua Sha for Digestive Health

Gua Sha is a therapy that has been used for centuries to improve digestive health and alleviate digestive symptoms. In this chapter, we will explore the benefits of Gua Sha for the digestive system, techniques to promote digestive health, and why the Sacred Healing Supply Company's Gua Sha tool is the perfect choice for promoting digestive health.

Benefits for the Digestive System

Gua Sha can help improve digestive health in a number of ways. It can help to:

- Reduce inflammation: Gua Sha can help to reduce inflammation in the digestive system, which can lead to improved digestion and a reduction in symptoms like bloating and cramping.
- Promote lymphatic drainage: By promoting lymphatic drainage, Gua Sha can help to remove excess fluid and

waste products from the digestive system, promoting better digestive function.

- Relieve tension: Gua Sha can help to relieve tension in the muscles and connective tissues surrounding the digestive system, which can help to improve digestion and reduce discomfort.

Techniques for Promoting Digestive Health

To promote digestive health with Gua Sha, it's important to use the right techniques. Here are some tips for promoting digestive health with Gua Sha:

- Start with a lubricant: Before using Gua Sha, it's important to apply a lubricant like oil or lotion to the skin. This will help the tool glide smoothly over the skin and reduce the risk of irritation or injury.
- Use gentle, sweeping strokes: When using Gua Sha for digestive health, use gentle, sweeping strokes to promote lymphatic drainage and reduce tension in the muscles and connective tissues surrounding the digestive system.
- Focus on specific areas: If you have specific areas of concern, such as bloating or discomfort, you can focus your Gua Sha treatment on those areas to promote better digestive function.

Why the Sacred Healing Supply Company's Gua Sha Tool is Perfect

The Sacred Healing Supply Company's Gua Sha tool is the perfect choice for promoting digestive health and improving the function of the digestive system. Its smooth, curved edges make it easy to use on the skin without causing discomfort, and the high-quality stainless steel construction ensures durability and long-lasting use. The tool can be used to gently scrape and massage the skin, promoting lymphatic drainage and reducing tension in the muscles and connective tissues surrounding the digestive system. Its ergonomic shape and smooth edges make it easy to use and comfortable to hold, even during longer sessions. Whether you're dealing with digestive issues like bloating or discomfort, the Sacred Healing Supply Company's Gua Sha tool is a reliable and effective choice for improving your digestive health and promoting better digestion.

In addition to Gua Sha, other lifestyle factors can also play a role in promoting digestive health. Eating a healthy, balanced diet, staying hydrated, and engaging in regular exercise can all contribute to better digestive function. By incorporating Gua Sha into your daily routine and focusing on other healthy lifestyle habits, you can enjoy better digestive health and improve your overall well-being.

In conclusion, Gua Sha can be an effective therapy for promoting digestive health and improving the function of the digestive system. By using the right techniques and incorporating the Sacred Healing Supply Company's Gua Sha tool into your daily self-care routine, you can enjoy the many benefits of Gua Sha and improve your digestive health naturally and effectively.

CHAPTER XI:

Gua Sha and Emotional Wellness

Gua Sha is a natural and non-invasive therapy that can help to improve both physical and emotional health. In this chapter, we will explore the connection between emotional and physical health, the benefits of Gua Sha for reducing stress and anxiety, techniques for promoting relaxation and improved mood, and why the Sacred Healing Supply Company's Gua Sha tool can help achieve those goals.

The Connection Between Emotional and Physical Health

There is a strong connection between emotional and physical health. When we experience emotional stress or anxiety, it can lead to physical symptoms like tension in the muscles, headaches, and digestive issues. Conversely, when we experience physical discomfort or pain, it can lead to emotional stress and anxiety. By using Gua Sha to improve physical health, we can also improve emotional well-being.

Techniques for Reducing Stress and Anxiety

Gua Sha can be a powerful tool for reducing stress and anxiety. Here are some techniques to try:

- Use a calming lubricant: Using a calming lubricant like lavender oil can help to promote relaxation and reduce stress during a Gua Sha session.
- Focus on specific areas: If you experience tension or discomfort in specific areas of the body, focusing your Gua Sha treatment on those areas can be particularly effective for reducing stress and anxiety.
- Use gentle, sweeping strokes: Using gentle, sweeping strokes with the Gua Sha tool can promote relaxation and reduce tension in the muscles and connective tissues.

Techniques for Promoting Relaxation and Improved Mood

Gua Sha can also be a powerful tool for promoting relaxation and an improved mood. Here are some techniques to try:

- Use a uplifting lubricant: Using an uplifting lubricant like bergamot or grapefruit oil can help to promote a positive mood and energy during a Gua Sha session.

- Focus on specific areas: If you have areas of the body that tend to hold tension, focusing your Gua Sha treatment on those areas can be particularly effective for promoting relaxation and an improved mood.
- Use gentle, sweeping strokes: Using gentle, sweeping strokes with the Gua Sha tool can help to promote relaxation and a sense of calm.

Why the Sacred Healing Supply Company's Gua Sha Tool is Perfect

The Sacred Healing Supply Company's Gua Sha tool is the perfect choice for improving emotional wellness. Its smooth, curved edges make it easy to use on the skin without causing discomfort, and the high-quality stainless steel construction ensures durability and long-lasting use. The tool can be used to gently scrape and massage the skin, promoting relaxation and reducing tension in the muscles and connective tissues. Its ergonomic shape and smooth edges make it easy to use and comfortable to hold, even during longer sessions.

By incorporating the Sacred Healing Supply Company's Gua Sha tool into your daily self-care routine, you can experience the many benefits of Gua Sha for emotional wellness. Whether you are experiencing stress, anxiety, or simply looking for a way to promote relaxation and an improved mood, Gua Sha can be a natural and effective solution.

In addition to Gua Sha, other lifestyle factors can also play a role in promoting emotional wellness. Engaging in regular exercise, practicing mindfulness and meditation, and seeking support from loved ones or a mental health professional can all contribute to better emotional health. By incorporating Gua Sha into your daily routine and focusing on other healthy lifestyle habits, you can enjoy better emotional wellness and improve your overall well-being.

In conclusion, Gua Sha can be a powerful tool for improving emotional wellness and promoting relaxation and an improved mood. By using the right techniques and incorporating the Sacred Healing Supply Company's Gua Sha tool into your daily self-care routine, you can experience the many benefits of Gua Sha and improve your emotional well-being naturally and effectively.

CHAPTER XII

Integrating Gua Sha Into a Wellness Routine

Gua Sha is a versatile and effective therapy that can complement a wide range of other wellness practices. In this chapter, we will explore how Gua Sha can be integrated into a wellness routine, tips for incorporating Gua Sha into a daily routine, frequently asked questions about Gua Sha, and why the Sacred Healing Supply Company's Gua Sha tool is the perfect choice for integrating Gua Sha into a wellness routine.

How Gua Sha Can Complement Other Wellness Practices

Gua Sha can complement a wide range of other wellness practices, including:

- Acupuncture: Gua Sha can be used in conjunction with acupuncture to enhance its effects and promote better overall health and wellness.

- Massage: Gua Sha can be used as a complementary therapy to massage, helping to promote relaxation and reduce tension in the muscles and connective tissues.
- Yoga and exercise: Gua Sha can be used to help prepare the body for yoga and exercise, promoting better circulation and reducing tension in the muscles.
- Skincare: Gua Sha can be used to promote better skin health and complement other skincare practices like facial massage and skincare products.

Tips for Incorporating Gua Sha into a Daily Routine

Here are some tips for incorporating Gua Sha into a daily routine:

- Start small: Begin by incorporating Gua Sha into your routine for just a few minutes each day, gradually increasing the length and frequency of your sessions over time.
- Choose a time of day that works for you: Whether you prefer to incorporate Gua Sha into your morning routine or before bed, choose a time that works for your schedule and lifestyle.
- Use Gua Sha as part of a self-care routine: Incorporate Gua Sha into a larger self-care routine that includes other healthy habits like exercise, healthy eating, and meditation.

Frequently Asked Questions About Gua Sha

Here are some frequently asked questions about Gua Sha:

- Is Gua Sha safe? Yes, Gua Sha is generally considered safe when performed properly. It's important to use a lubricant to avoid irritation or injury, and to be mindful of any areas of the body that may be more sensitive or prone to bruising.
- Is Gua Sha painful? Gua Sha should not be painful, but some people may experience a mild discomfort or sensation of warmth during the treatment.
- How often should I do Gua Sha? The frequency of Gua Sha treatments can vary depending on your needs and preferences. Some people may choose to do Gua Sha daily, while others may choose to incorporate it into their routine a few times a week.

Why the Sacred Healing Supply Company's Gua Sha Tool is Perfect

The Sacred Healing Supply Company's Gua Sha tool is the perfect choice for integrating Gua Sha into a wellness routine. Its smooth, curved edges make it easy to use on the skin without causing discomfort, and the high-quality stainless steel construction ensures durability and long-lasting use. The tool can be used to gently scrape and massage the skin, promoting relaxation and reducing tension in the muscles and connective tissues. Its ergonomic shape and smooth edges make it easy to use and comfortable to hold, even during longer sessions.

By incorporating the Sacred Healing Supply Company's Gua Sha tool into your daily self-care routine, you can experience the many benefits of Gua Sha and improve your overall health and wellness. Whether you're looking to promote relaxation, reduce tension in the muscles, or improve skin health, Gua Sha can be a powerful tool for achieving your wellness goals.

In conclusion, Gua Sha can be a versatile and effective therapy that can complement a wide range of other wellness practices. By incorporating Gua Sha into your daily routine and focusing on other healthy lifestyle habits, you can enjoy the many benefits of Gua Sha and improve your overall well-being. With the tips and techniques provided in this book, as well as the use of the Sacred Healing Supply Company's Gua Sha tool, you can easily integrate this therapy into your wellness routine and experience the many benefits it has to offer.

Remember, it's important to be mindful of your body's needs and limitations when incorporating any new wellness practice. If you have any concerns or questions about Gua Sha, be sure to consult with a healthcare provider before beginning a new routine.

In summary, Gua Sha is a natural and non-invasive therapy with numerous benefits for the body and mind. Whether you're seeking pain relief, improved skin health, or emotional well-being, Gua Sha can be a powerful tool for achieving your wellness goals. With the information provided in this book and the use of the Sacred Healing Supply Company's Gua Sha tool, you can easily integrate this therapy into your daily self-care routine and enjoy the many benefits it has to offer.

The Sacred Healing Supply Company's Gua Sha tool is not only a perfect choice for incorporating Gua Sha into a wellness routine, but it also complements other wellness practices like the Infrared Red Light Therapy Belt. The combination of these two therapies can enhance the overall effectiveness of your wellness routine, promoting better circulation, relaxation, and pain relief.

The Infrared Red Light Therapy Belt can be used to target specific areas of the body, while the Gua Sha tool can be used to promote lymphatic drainage and reduce tension in the muscles and connective tissues. Together, these therapies can help to alleviate pain, reduce inflammation, and promote better overall health and wellness.

Both the Sacred Healing Supply Company's Gua Sha tool and Infrared Red Light Therapy Belt are available for purchase on our website, as well as on Amazon and other fine retailers. By using these tools in combination, you can create a comprehensive and effective wellness routine that promotes optimal health and well-being. Whether you're seeking pain relief, improved skin health, or emotional well-being, these tools can help you achieve your wellness goals.

So, whether you're a seasoned practitioner of natural wellness or you're just starting out, the Sacred Healing Supply Company's Gua Sha tool and Infrared Red Light Therapy Belt are the perfect tools to help you improve your overall well-being. Try them out today and experience the many benefits they have to offer.

About the Authors

Michael DiCicco and Estrella Ortega are co-founders of the Sacred Healing Supply Company, a leading provider of natural wellness tools and accessories. With a shared passion for natural health and wellness, Michael and Estrella have dedicated their careers to helping people live healthier, happier, and more fulfilling lives.

Michael DiCicco is a lifelong entrepreneur with a deep interest in natural health and wellness. After struggling with chronic pain for years, Michael discovered the power of Gua Sha and other natural therapies to alleviate his symptoms and improve his overall well-being. Inspired by his own experiences, he founded the Sacred Healing Supply Company to share these tools with others and promote natural healing and wellness.

Estrella Ortega is a wellness expert and Gua Sha practitioner with over a decade of experience in the natural health industry. After witnessing the transformative power of Gua Sha in her own life and the lives of her clients, Estrella joined forces with Michael to bring these natural healing tools to a wider audience. She is passionate about sharing the benefits of Gua Sha and other natural therapies with others and helping them achieve optimal health and wellness.

In addition to their work with the Sacred Healing Supply Company, Michael and Estrella are also the authors of "The Sacred Healing Light: Unlocking the Power of Infrared Red Light Therapy for Humans and Pets." This book explores the many benefits of infrared therapy for both people and animals, and provides practical tips and advice for incorporating this therapy into your wellness routine.

Together, Michael and Estrella bring a wealth of knowledge and experience to the field of natural health and wellness. They are dedicated to providing high-quality products, resources, and information to help people live happier, healthier, and more fulfilling lives. Through their work as authors and entrepreneurs, they are helping to transform the way people approach health and wellness, one person at a time.

About Sacred Healing Supply Company

"Honoring tradition, embracing innovation" - Sacred Healing Supply Company

At Sacred Healing Supply Company, we believe that technology and ancient wisdom can work together to promote healing and well-being. Our mission is to provide individuals with the latest in cutting-edge technology and traditional spiritual tools and resources. We strive to empower people to take an active role in their own healing journey by offering a wide range of products and services that integrate technology and spiritual practices. Our goal is to create a sense of balance and harmony in people's lives by combining the best of both worlds and helping people access the power of the sacred and the benefits of technology to promote physical, emotional, and spiritual well-being.

For More Information and Access to Our Great Products, head over to www.SacredHealingSupply.com

Copyright Disclaimer:

The information presented in this book is based on the authors' personal experiences and research and is not intended to be a comprehensive guide to Gua Sha or natural health and wellness. The authors make no representations or warranties of any kind, express or implied, about the completeness, accuracy, reliability, suitability, or availability of the information contained in this book. Any reliance you place on such information is strictly at your own risk.

The authors and the Sacred Healing Supply Company are not liable for any direct or indirect consequences of the use of Gua Sha or any other natural therapy. Always use Gua Sha safely and with caution, and discontinue use if you experience any adverse reactions or discomfort. It is important to do your own research and consult with a qualified healthcare provider before making any changes to your wellness routine.